Weight Loss
30 Days to a Slimmer, Leaner and Beautiful Body

Table of Contents

Introduction

You have more than likely heard time and time again about how important it is for you to lose weight. You've probably heard stories about the benefits of losing weight while also noticing just how unappealing you might be if you weighed more than necessary.

The added cost of medical services when you're overweight can be a problem. The threat of added health risks can especially be serious. The fact that you won't look as great to other people as you might wish you could be will especially be a cause for concern.

But how do you go about losing weight?

Better yet, how can you do so in a shorter period of time? This guide will help you understand everything you can do when trying to lose weight. This will guide you through a setup to help you lose weight and feel your best in 30 days. The results that will come about from this guide will vary. You will still have a healthier and more positive body after using this guide for 30 days. You'll not only have lost some weight but you will also be on the right path with some healthy routines and dietary habits to help you keep losing weight well after that first 30 day period.

It is not as complicated for you to lose weight as you might think it could be either. As you will see in this guide, there are many things that go into the process of losing weight that deserve to be explored in detail.

You will learn in this guide about how you can get motivated to lose weight and how you can avoid many of the difficult habits in your life that might keep you from losing weight. You will also learn about how exercise and nutritional strategies can assist you in losing weight.

The points listed in this guide are detailed enough to help you make the most out of your weight loss plan. Even with this, they are still easy enough to where it won't be all that hard for you to follow the rules for weight loss that you will read about here.

Get ready to have fun with losing weight and feeling better about your body. You might be surprised at what you will get out of yourself. Better yet, you might start to think that you should be used the points in this guide a little sooner.

Chapter 1 – Getting Motivated

The first thing you have to do when looking to lose weight is to find a way to be motivated. It is often a challenge for you to lose weight because you might not feel much of a need for doing so.

The fact is that there are more than enough reasons why you need to lose weight. It's about giving yourself a body you will be more comfortable with or to keep yourself from being at a serious risk of various substantial and dangerous medical issues. It's also about giving yourself a more energetic and productive life as you will have more energy when you lose weight and feel better about your body.

Getting motivated is just the first step towards getting that body you have always dreamed about. There are many things that can be done to motivate you to lose weight and get started on the road to a healthy life.

Prepare a Goal

The first thing to do is to figure out your goal for losing weight. A sensible goal should be established to help you figure out how you're going to lose weight and run a routine that is sensible and easy to follow.

There are many goals that you can consider:

- You can find a way to cut down on your caloric intake. A pound typically equals about 3,500 calories. Getting rid of about 500 calories in a day is always a good goal to set up at the start.
- Consider your wardrobe and think about anything you wear that might not fit as well as it used to. You could always make it a goal for you to lose enough weight to where you can actually fit in those outfits again.

- Set up a round number in terms of the weight total you want to be at. Try to keep that round number from being more than 20 pounds lighter than what you are, for instance. If you weigh 218 pounds then you can set up a goal of 200 pounds.

The best thing to do here is to talk with a doctor to see what you could get out of a goal. Your doctor may take a look at points like your body type, your medical history and so forth. It could all help you to lose weight in a safe and sensible manner.

Work With Someone

It is often easier for you to lose weight if you are motivated by others who are working with the same goals as you are. Working out and living a healthier lifestyle with other people who want to lose weight is great for a variety of reasons:
- You can make friends with others who have a goal similar to yours.
- You can compete with others to see who can get the most out of their weight loss plans.
- It might help to get pointers and ideas from others who want to lose weight. Sharing ideas and plans always helps when it comes to figuring out what you can do to lose weight.

Check to see if there are people at your place of employment who might be working hard to lose weight. Look for weight loss classes in your area as well as they might be held by different health care centers or gyms. The odds are there is something in your area that you can take advantage of when learning to lose weight with other people.

The best part of working with someone else while losing weight is that you will be prepared to work a little harder when you do so with another person. You might be amazed at how motivational it can be for you to lose weight with other people.

Start a Blog or Journal

A simple blog or journal can be a rather motivational tool. This could help you to keep track of what you are doing from a weight loss perspective.

You can use a journal to help you keep track of what you have been doing when trying to lose weight. It can include points on your dietary and exercise activities for the day as well as any supplements you might have taken.

This could help you keep track of how well you are losing weight. It may also help you to figure out what you are doing right or what needs to change for you to actively lose weight. The process of motivation does not have to be a real challenge to handle. Make sure you follow the right rules when finding ways to get ready to lose weight.

Chapter 2 – Avoiding Old Habits

To actually lose weight, you have to watch out for how you are going to go about with losing it in a sensible manner. Part of this includes making sure you avoid the old habits that might have caused you to gain weight or at least keep you from losing weight.

What Are the Most Common Bad Habits?

There are many habits that keep people from losing weight properly. These include such habits as the following problems:

- You're not getting the sleep you need.

- You often go shopping for food when you're hungry.

- You consume foods without thinking about what you're putting into your body.

- You may also skip important meals.

This chapter is devoted to helping you understand some of the bad habits you might get yourself into. This also delves into how you can avoid getting into the habits that cause you to gain weight or at least struggle to lose it.

Don't Stay Up So Much

The first thing to do is to avoid staying up as late you might have in the past. Staying awake for longer than necessary can prove to be a real problem. A lack of sleep will keep your body from producing cortisol, a critical hormone that controls your appetite.

In addition, your body will be more likely to store fat when you don't get enough sleep. This in turn makes it harder for you to actually lose weight. Getting a better night's sleep is a necessity for when you need to keep yourself under control.

Avoid Shopping When Hungry

One of the biggest reasons why people often spend more money on groceries is because they shop while hungry. To make things worse, people often pick up the first things they see when they are hungry. This is regardless of how unhealthy certain foods might be.

You need to eat something healthy before you go outside the house. This is to keep you from being at risk of buying things that you know are unhealthy for you, whether it is at a local grocery store or at some other place that offers various foods.

Avoid Whatever Might Be Convenient

We always look for foods that are convenient. These include things packaged in bars, wraps and other things that you can open up and eat with ease. But that doesn't mean those foods are actually good for all of us.

The problem with many foods that might seem convenient is that they are actually more harmful for our bodies than we think. Many foods that are packaged with convenience in mind are ones that are dangerous to our bodies because they contain lots of fillers, preservatives and other ingredients that keep us from being healthy.

The lack of healthy things in these foods can cause anyone to gain weight. This could be a real threat to your body if not used right.

Avoid Skipping Breakfast

It's often easy for anyone to skip breakfast. You might be guilty of doing so on the basis that you are in a hurry for whatever reason.

Your body needs a healthy meal at the start of the day to help your metabolic rate improve over time. You need to get something healthy to start yourself up right so your body can burn off fat and get enough energy to make it through a typical day.

Skipping breakfast is dangerous in that it keeps you from burning calories and fats. It keeps your body from being able to keep its metabolic processes running. Therefore, you have to always have a good breakfast and avoid the habit of skipping it.

Don't Use the Wrong Portions

The last thing that causes people to gain weight involves portion sizes. We take portion sizes for granted these days. We think that a larger portion is normal and that we can consume such big portions. However, this mindset is dangerous as you could end up eating more than what your body can handle.

You have to avoid going after the massive portions of foods that might be available to you in a typical day. You have to keep your foods from being too big or otherwise difficult to handle.

Be sure to watch for the habits that you get into when trying to lose weight. You have to avoid the bad habits that might have caused you to gain weight or have kept you from burning it off.

Chapter 3 – Nutrients That Trigger Weight Loss

It's clear that you need to have a healthy diet if you want to lose weight. However, you can't just eat anything to lose weight.

Having a sensible amount of food each day is important. You clearly need to keep from consuming more calories in a typical day than what you might be used to. Still, the nutrients in the foods that you eat will make a difference when you're trying to lose weight.

This chapter is all about the nutrients that you need to consume in your diet in order to lose weight. This will be followed up by a 30-day plan that you can utilize with many foods that entail the healthy foods.

What makes the nutrients listed here important is that they will assist in the fat-burning process. This is the most crucial aspect of weight loss that you should consider as it helps improve how well your body functions over time.

Many of these nutrients can also control your appetite. Some of these will even improve how well you can manage water in your body so you don't store more water than necessary.

Arginine

Arginine is an amino acid that will help you with losing weight. It is an amino acid that controls how visceral adipose fat, or belly fat as it is often called, is taken into the body. It prevents new fats from developing in that region.

This improves lipolysis, a process where fatty acids are burned off, and improves how blood vessels function. It particular dilates those blood vessels, what with arginine being a precursor to nitric oxide. As this works, the heart will have an easier time pumping blood and delivering the nutrients your body needs all around.

Arginine is typically found in a variety of great foods:

- Lean beef, particularly grass-fed beef

- Lean chicken

- Various nuts including almonds, walnuts and peanuts

- Eggs

- Assorted dairy products including milk and cheese

- Oats and various other forms of whole wheat

Potassium

Potassium is often associated with bananas, one of the easiest fruits for anyone to eat. There are many other foods besides bananas that feature potassium though.

The key part of potassium is that it keeps your body energetic. It improves upon how you can recover after a workout. It helps you to clear water and sodium out of your body, thus keeping you from bearing with water weight that makes you tire out easily. In return, the bloating that you might experience on occasion will be reduced or eliminated.

Potassium also helps to improve how the kidneys function. It especially keeps the kidneys from wearing out as it improves how they can clear water waste.

Obviously, the banana is a very popular food to have when you need potassium. There are plenty of other great foods to have when you're looking for this important mineral:

- Leafy green vegetables

- Molasses

- Avocados

- Various nuts

Magnesium

Magnesium is a mineral that is critical to your body's health. This assists in the production of natural muscular functions that work within your body. It especially assists in promoting muscle contractions. As a result, proteins will be processed with ease, thus improving how well you can burn off fats. Also, magnesium helps to reduce your fasting glucose and insulin levels. These levels are important as high glucose and insulin levels can cause you to store more fat in your body. Magnesium also improves upon the lipolysis process. This in turn releases fats from all around your body, thus improving how well your body will stay healthy.

There are many great foods that contain magnesium:

- Nuts, particularly almonds

- Leafy green vegetables, especially spinach

- Various beans

- Whole grains including whole wheat bread and brown rice

Resistant Starch

Starch is a commonplace compound found in many grains. Starch might be useful for keeping you full and ready for a typical day but it might not be all that great for weight loss. The problem with traditional starch is that it can stay in your digestive tract for a while. This makes it harder for the tract to be cleared out. It is also harder for the body to take in the nutrients it requires for weight loss.

This is where resistant starch can come into play. This is a type of starch known as slow carbs. This works in that it moves through your small intestine without being digested. As it moves through the digestive tract without any obstructions, it improves upon the production of healthy gut bacteria.

That gut bacteria is needed to improve how your body's digestive functions work. This assists in burning off fat while giving your body a fuller feeling for a longer period of time. This in turn enhances how you can lose weight.

Resistant starch is important in that it does not break down to where it can get in the way of your body's natural digestive functions. This can certainly be easier for you to consume than traditional starches that might not be as well-refined as they should be.

There are plenty of resistant starch options to look for in your diet. Here are some of the better choices for you to add:

- Raw potatoes

- Cooked and cooled potatoes

- Green bananas

- Raw oats

- Various beans

- Raw barley

Leucine

There is a need for your body to properly manage the protein it is getting. Leucine is one particular nutrient that will help.

Leucine is an amino acid that improves how proteins are consumed by the body. By using leucine, proteins are properly synthesized to where your metabolic rate will go up. This in turn improves how well you can lose weight. By keeping that rate up, more fats and calories can be burned at a more efficient rate.

There are many good sources of leucine to look for:

- Chicken, particularly chicken breast

- Eggs

- Fish

- Lean beef and pork

Vitamin D

Vitamin D has long been heralded as a popular vitamin that will help you with improve your bone structure. When used with calcium, it improves upon the formation of natural bone cells in your body. This in turn gives you a stronger and sturdier body while preventing potential fractures and breakages from developing.

This is great in its own right but there's more to vitamin D than you think. It may also be used as a great vitamin for your weight loss requirements.

Vitamin D regulates your appetite and your hunger. This improves how well you eat foods so you won't be at risk of eating more than necessary.

This is also known to control how belly fat develops. It improves how well belly fat breaks down and keeps new fats from developing. Considering how challenging this kind of fat might be for you to burn off, it is a necessity to see what you can do when trying to keep it from being all that problematic.

Vitamin D is naturally found in a variety of great foods. Naturally, fortified dairy products like cheese and milk products are always great to have. However, it might also help to add a few extras to your routine.

These are some of the best foods to consider when looking for things that have enough vitamin D for your body:

- Tuna, mackerel and other fatty fish with oil

- Beef liver

- Eggs, particularly their yolks

- Various foods fortified with vitamin D; these include cereals, orange juice and more

- Some soy-based dairy substitutes may be fortified with vitamin D although they might not contain as much of it as other dairy-based items

Naturally, vitamin D can be produced within the body as you are exposed to the sun's rays. However, you cannot rely on that vitamin D alone. You have to get enough healthy foods with vitamin D into your body to give yourself the added support you deserve. In addition, you would clearly have to use enough sun protectant materials and lotions around your skin if you were to try and get enough of this vitamin from the sun.

Monounsaturated Fats

Not all fats are created equal. Monounsaturated fats are among the best fats to have for your weight loss needs.

These fats are ones that become solid as they are chilled. In particular, the fat molecules have one unsaturated carbon bond each. This is what causes the fat to go from being a liquid while at room temperature to solid when it gets a little colder.

These fats may help with improving how well your body burns off other fats. Monounsaturated fats will break down quite well and trigger other fats to start burning off. This in turn makes you feel a little healthier and stronger. If used right, it will improve how well you are able to keep your body healthy.

The foods that are high in monounsaturated fat that will do well for your diet include:

- Olives

- Macadamia nuts

- Peanut butter

- Coconuts

- Dark chocolate

- Grass-fed beef

Oils relating to the foods listed here may also work for your diet. These oils will help you out by giving you the necessary support demanded for keeping your body healthy.

Like with any other fat out there, you have to be cautious when using these. An excess amount of any kind of fat can still cause you to gain weight.

Omega-3 Fatty Acids

We have all heard about omega-3 fatty acids these days to the point where it's practically a buzzword. The fact is that omega-3 fatty acids are ideal for your weight loss needs in that they contain the right amounts of healthy compounds to help you lose weight and keep it off.

These fatty acids are typically found in fish oil and are capable of triggering many healthy functions in your body. They will start by improving how blood moves throughout the body. This is clearly to get key nutrients to move around your body. Omega-3 fatty acids also stimulate the production of enzymes that move fats to different parts of the body where they can be used up. These fats are released as they are burned off for use as energy. This in turn creates a healthier body over time. These fatty acids may also improve how well your brain functions and keep the risk of strokes and other serious problems from developing. Further research is needed to determine for certain if these fatty acids are as useful for this purpose as they are said to be.

The foods to find when getting omega-3 fatty acids clearly entail fish, what with the oils from these fish naturally having them. It is best to have wild fish and not farmed ones as farmed fish are typically less likely to have omega-3s. This is due to farmed fish being treated with many outside compounds and put under enough stress to where their healthy fats will quickly be lost over time.

Also, salmon is the most popular fish to look for when finding omega-3 fatty acids. Other fish options like tuna and halibut may also work. Again, these should be fresh and wild.

There are plenty of other foods besides fish that contain omega-3 fatty acids:

- Eggs; look for ones that are enriched with omega-3s

- Grass-fed lean beef; anything prepared with outside chemicals might be harmful

- Flaxseed oil

- Various nuts, particularly walnuts

Fruits and Vegetables

It's clear that there are plenty of fine grains, meats and other things that can help you out with getting your weight loss goals under control. But what about fruits and vegetables? It's always a good idea to have fruits and vegetables in your diet. These all contain plenty of healthy nutrients and fewer calories than many other foods. You can also get fiber off of these foods to improve how you manage your appetite.
Still, all fruits and vegetables are varied. Here are a few good options to consider when finding ones for your weight loss needs. These are organized based on the total amount that is appropriate for an average serving:

- A single traditional fruit like a banana, apple and orange

- Half an avocado or grapefruit

- A few kiwi fruits or plums

- 3 teaspoons of beans of varying forms

- A single traditional vegetable like a celery stalk or carrot

- One cup of berries or grapes

- A large pineapple or melon slice

- A glass of juice pressed from any of these fruits or vegetables; this might be best as it is easier for you to digest this type of juice

These are designed primarily to help control your appetite and to keep you from eating more than necessary. By using enough fruits and vegetables, it will be easier for you to manage your appetite without risking any serious harm to how your diet is running.

It is impressive to see how all of these foods can help you with getting more out of your weight loss goals. These are all made with more than enough healthy vitamins and nutrients that trigger weight loss functions.

Chapter 4 – 30 Days of the Right Foods

Now that you have a clear idea of what nutrients will work out right for your body, it is time to take a look at a 30-day plan to help you lose weight. This 30-day plan focuses on the three basic meals of the day to make it easier for you to keep your metabolic functions up and running.

You'll also notice that every day comes with an option for you to have a between-meal snack. This includes something that should be easy for your body to take in.

The portions used in this guide should also be good enough for your body to handle. These are sensible in that you will get enough of a meal each time without forcing yourself to take in more calories than necessary.

Day 1
Breakfast: 1 orange and a bowl of whole grain cereal
Lunch: 2 ounces fruit salad, particularly with diced melons, pineapples and apples
Dinner: 3 ounces lean beef
Optional In-Between Meal: 1 ounce walnuts

Day 2
Breakfast: 1 egg with a bowl of whole grain cereal
Lunch: 2 ounces tuna with whole wheat crackers
Dinner: 4 ounces grilled chicken breast
Optional In-Between Meal: 1 glass of milk and a fresh 1-ounce slice of cheese

Day 3
Breakfast: 3 links lean turkey sausage
Lunch: 2 ounces leafy greens with diced peanuts and cashews
Dinner: 4 ounces spinach and kale with olive oil and diced olives
Optional In-Between Meal: ¼ ounce dark chocolate

Day 4
Breakfast: 2 egg whites

Lunch: 2 to 3 ounces of spinach mixed with ¼-cup avocado
Dinner: 3 ounces grilled turkey with a raw potato
Optional In-Between Meal: 8 ounces of fresh pressed carrot juice

Day 5
Breakfast: 1 bowl of whole grain cereal plus 6 ounces of vitamin D-enriched soy milk
Lunch: 2 ounces lean chicken breast with 3 carrot sticks
Dinner: 2 ounces lean grass-fed beef and 2 ounces black beans in a whole wheat flour tortilla; this may be used as a burrito
Optional In-Between Meal: 2 ounces pressed wheatgrass juice

Day 6
Breakfast: 1 egg
Lunch: 2 ounces lean turkey sausage with 2 ounces whole grain brown rice and black beans
Dinner: 4 ounces spinach and kale with sprinkled berries and nuts
Optional In-Between Meal: Half an ounce molasses on two slices of whole wheat toast

Day 7
Breakfast: 1 apple and 1 orange
Lunch: Half an avocado spread on whole wheat toast
Dinner: 2 ounces salmon with half a raw potato
Optional In-Between Meal: 1 cup of red grapes

Day 8
Breakfast: 1 egg and 2 links of lean chicken sausage
Lunch: 1 ounce chicken breast between two slices of whole wheat bread
Dinner:
Optional In-Between Meal: 1 cup blueberries

Day 9
Breakfast: 2 eggs and 1 turkey sausage

Lunch: 2 ounces tuna with 1 ounce baked beans
Dinner: 4 ounces spinach and kale with 1 ounce grilled chicken
Optional In-Between Meal: 1 cup whole grain popcorn

Day 10
Breakfast: 1 bowl whole grain cereal
Lunch: 2 ounces salmon and half a tomato
Dinner: 3 ounces lean beef with a whole grain roll
Optional In-Between Meal: 1 cup strawberries

Day 11
Breakfast: 2 ounces strawberries and a full banana
Lunch: 2 ounces ham with one pineapple ring
Dinner: 2 ounces salmon with 2 ounces lettuce
Optional In-Between Meal: 1 or 2 pineapple slices

Day 12
Breakfast: 2 ounces strawberries with plain yogurt
Lunch: 2 ounces lima beans and 2 ounces peas mixed with a diced carrot
Dinner: 3 ounces crayfish with 2 Portobello mushrooms
Optional In-Between Meal: 1 ounce peanuts

Day 13
Breakfast: 2 eggs and 2 links of turkey sausage
Lunch: 3 or 4 sardines with whole grain toast
Dinner: 2 ounces lean ham with two pineapple slices
Optional In-Between Meal: 1 ounce macadamia nuts

Day 14
Breakfast: 1 full banana and half a cup of yogurt
Lunch: 2 ounce squash with diced apples
Dinner: 3 ounces cabbage with 2 ounces boiled salmon
Optional In-Between Meal: 2 or 3 plums

Day 15

Breakfast: 1 bowl whole grain cereal
Lunch: 2 ounces romaine lettuce and 1 diced tomato
Dinner: 3 ounces white turkey breast and 1 sweet potato
Optional In-Between Meal: 4 to 6 prunes

Day 16
Breakfast: 2 ounces blueberries with plain yogurt
Lunch: 2 celery stalks and 1 carrot with whole grain chips
Dinner: 2 ounces whole grain brown rice with 1 diced turkey sausage
Optional In-Between Meal: 1 or 2 ounces grapefruit

Day 17
Breakfast: 1 bowl of whole grain cereal with 8 ounces of vitamin D-enriched orange juice
Lunch: 1 sliced lean sausage with 2 ounces black beans and 2 ounces brown rice
Dinner: 2 ounces cooked salmon with 2 ounces lettuce
Optional In-Between Meal: 1 banana or orange

Day 18
Breakfast: 1 bowl of whole oat oatmeal; look for steel cut oats if possible
Lunch: 2 ounces ground bison meat on two whole wheat buns
Dinner: 3 ounces lettuce mixed with 2 ounces strawberries and half a celery stalk
Optional In-Between Meal: 3 teaspoons black beans; these can be mashed and used with whole grain chips if desired

Day 19
Breakfast: 2 ounces blueberries with about 2 ounces yogurt
Lunch: 2 ounces grilled chicken with 2 ounces black beans
Dinner: 3 ounces grilled salmon
Optional In-Between Meal: 1 cup whole grain popcorn

Day 20
Breakfast: 3 ounces fruit salad with diced items

Lunch: 2 ounces cooked chicken breast
Dinner: 2 ounces grass-fed lean beef with 2 ounces broccoli
Optional In-Between Meal: 1 slice of whole wheat toast with olive oil

Day 21
Breakfast: Half a pitted mango with a bowl of cereal
Lunch: 2 ounces ground bison and 2 slices whole wheat toast
Dinner: 3 ounces salmon with half a raw potato
Optional In-Between Meal: 2 ounces whole grain chips

Day 22
Breakfast: 2 or 3 diced figs
Lunch: 2 ounces romaine lettuce plus one ounce kale
Dinner: 3 ounces grilled salmon with three asparagus stalks
Optional In-Between Meal: 2 ounces wheatgrass juice

Day 23
Breakfast: 2 ounces yogurt with crushed walnuts
Lunch: 2 slices whole grain toast with 2 or 3 sardines
Dinner: 2 ounces lean beef with one diced pepper
Optional In-Between Meal: 1 slice whole wheat toast with olive oil

Day 24
Breakfast: 2 ounces watermelon with one apple
Lunch: 2 ounces grilled chicken
Dinner: 2 ounces soft shell crab meat with half a tomato
Optional In-Between Meal: 1 ounce whole grain popcorn

Day 25
Breakfast: 1 bowl of whole oat oatmeal
Lunch: 2 ounces garden peas mixed with 2 ounces grilled chicken
Dinner: 1 cob of corn and 2 ounces of baked salmon
Optional In-Between Meal: 1/4 ounce dark chocolate

Day 26
Breakfast: 2 ounces grapes and a slice of whole wheat toast
Lunch: 2 ounces green beans mixed with 1 tomato
Dinner: 3 ounces tuna with half a tomato
Optional In-Between Meal: 1 cup of yogurt with berries of your choice

Day 27
Breakfast: 2 ounces yogurt with diced strawberries and raspberries
Lunch: 2 ounces sardines with half a tomato
Dinner: 1 sweet potato and 2 ounces kale
Optional In-Between Meal: 2 ounces whole grain chips

Day 28
Breakfast: 1 bowl of whole oat oatmeal with 1 ounces blueberries
Lunch: 3 ounces ground lean beef with two whole wheat buns
Dinner: 3 ounces broiled catfish with 2 ounces sweet potatoes
Optional In-Between Meal: 1 ounce wheatgrass juice

Day 29
Breakfast: 2 ounces strawberries and a slice of whole grain toast
Lunch: Half a raw potato with 2 ounces blueberries
Dinner: 3 ounces lean beef with half a sweet potato
Optional In-Between Meal: 4 to 6 prunes

Day 30
Breakfast: 2 cups yogurt and one egg
Lunch: 1 sweet potato and 2 ounces lettuce
Dinner: 3 ounces rainbow trout and 2 ounces whole grain brown rice
Optional In-Between Meal: 2 ounces whole grain chips

Chapter 5 – What Supplements Work?

There's no such thing as a magical pill that lets you lose weight no matter what happens. If there was then there would be no need for this guide. However, there are a few supplements that may help you out with your weight loss needs.

These supplements are made with a variety of compounds that will make it easier for your body to benefit from the weight loss process. These are to be paired with a healthy diet and exercise routine to enhance how well you can lose weight. The added amount of weight that may be lost will vary by how well you respond to the product. You may get a few extra pounds off your body on a 30-day period. It might be one or two or even five pounds but every pound matters.

The supplements that are listed in this chapter are designed to be used on a regular basis. When taken properly, they will add more to your weight loss plans as they simply make it easier for you to lose weight.

Be advised that the dosage for each option will vary based on the instructions listed on a bottle for any of these products.

Garcinia Cambogia

Garcinia Cambogia is a pumpkin-shaped fruit that has been in the news in recent time. Its skin contains HCA or hydroxycitric acid. This compound stops enzymes that produce fats from functioning as well as they should.

This in turn improves how well you can burn off existing fats. It keeps any fats that are consumed in a healthy diet from being worse than they could be. It could help you lose a few extra pounds in 30 days.

This does not cause any serious side effects either. It might cause digestive issues in some people though.

Caffeine

A mild caffeine supplement can be ideal for your use. Caffeine is naturally found in tea, chocolate and coffee products. This does more than just improve how well your body might keep itself alert. It can also improve metabolic functions.
A caffeine supplement that works on its own without anything that contains sugar will improve how well your body's metabolic processes work. This in turn makes it easier for your body to burn off more calories and fats.
You will have to be careful when getting this supplement to work for you. Some supplements can cause you to develop feelings of irritability, restlessness and even diarrhea. Be very careful as you use this supplement.

Raspberry Ketones

Berries are great for your body as they provide you with fiber and can keep you from being too hungry throughout the day. However, there is more to berries than you might think. The raspberry in particular is a powerful one in that it features raspberry ketones.
Raspberry ketones are found in the raspberry and are substances that cause these berries to develop a distinctive scent. These can also break down fat cells and burn them off quite well.
In particular, these ketones also increase the levels of adiponectin in the body. This is a hormone that triggers weight loss functions by improving how the body's metabolic processes work.
As these fat cells break down, you will start to lose a little more weight. This in turn improves how well your body is able to respond to weight loss.

This might take a bit to work as your body gets used to the consumption of such ketones. However, regular use of such ketones can help you burn off fat cells quite well, thus giving you an added boost to your weight loss routine.

Green Coffee Bean Extract

Green coffee beans are beans that have not been roasted yet. You obviously cannot drink coffee made from these beans as you'd have to roast them to do this. However, the extracts that come from these coffee beans can be used in a supplement that will be to your weight loss benefit.

Green coffee beans contain chlorogenic acid. This is a component that is lost as you brew coffee beans. This acid will slow down how carbohydrates are broken down in your body. This keeps you from consuming more food than necessary.

This extract may assist in reducing your blood sugar levels and blood pressure totals. It may also clear out oxygen particles that might make it harder for you to stay healthy and energetic.

This is a great product for your weight loss needs but it may come with some of the same side effects as caffeine. You must see how well your body can tolerate this before committing to it; this might entail a need to consume less of this extract at the start.

Green Tea Extract

The next option to see is green tea extract. This is a popular product for weight loss use in that it also speeds up your metabolic processes.

Green tea extract comes from the leaves used to make green tea. The extract contains compounds that improve upon the production of norepinephrine. This hormone triggers fat-burning processes in your body.

This is easy to tolerate and will improve upon your fat-burning functions. Still, it does have a bit of caffeine in it. Make sure your body can tolerate caffeine before you try using this.

Bitter Orange

Bitter orange is a component that will release synephrine in your body. This is an ephedrine-like compound that is safer for you to handle than the actual ephedrine compound, a weight loss product that has been outlawed due to its serious side effects.

Bitter orange, a prominent plant, is not as potent as real ephedrine but it will reduce your appetite and improve how well your body can burn off fats. This is a good stimulant that is easy for your body to tolerate. Still, you should start off small to see that it won't be any harder for you to consume than necessary.

Be sure to talk with your doctor about any supplement that you want to use beforehand. Remember that everyone will respond to these supplements differently. Those who can respond to them well can certainly get more out of a weight loss plan when the right dietary plan is used alongside these supplements.

Chapter 6 – Mental Strategies For Life

As you read earlier in this guide, you have to avoid the many mental mistakes that can cause you to gain weight or struggle with your weight loss. This chapter is about a different point – it is about using the right mental strategies to help you keep going in your effort to lose weight and keep it off.

Create Smaller Goals

The key goal is to lose weight in 30 days. You should not be too vast in terms of your goal though.
The key is to create smaller goals that might be easier for you to maintain. These smaller goals are important as they help you keep a good pace to get to some of the larger goals over time.
You might want to utilize a goal of losing 5 pounds in about 30 days, for instance. You can then set a goal of losing 5 more pounds in another 30 days. This could give you a little more control over how you're going to lose weight.
The smaller goals that you set up will help you to get more out of your life. This is thanks to how you won't have to worry about any significant struggles with trying to reach particular goals that might be a little too hard for you to follow.

Work With Others

It is always a great idea to work with other people when you're aiming to lose weight. A great idea would be for you to exercise with other people who are trying to lose weight and to meet with others who are on their own weight loss programs.

Meeting with other people is always a great idea to consider. This helps you get in touch with other people so you can compare ideas and plans for weight loss with one another. This makes it easier for you to have a healthier lifestyle as you know that you're working with others to lose weight.

You can always hire a dietician to help you out as well. This is provided that you can afford the service. A dietician is a person who will help you out by providing you with advice and guidance for your weight loss plans. The solutions that your dietician can provide you with should help you to get the most out of what you want to do when losing weight.

Watch Your Portions

One of the main reasons why so many people gain weight comes from how they are unable to handle the portions of the foods they are trying to eat. In particular, people often eat more food than necessary because they don't know when to stop.

You have to watch out when you are trying to enjoy a good meal. You should not order portions that are any larger than they really have to be. In particular, you need to order portions that are suitable and small to keep you from eating more before your body knows when to stop.

A great tip is to use smaller plates and materials for eating. This will keep you from adding more food than necessary, what with there being a limit in terms of what you can add to your meal. This in turn keeps you from thinking that it is a good idea for you to consume more food than whatever it is that you can really handle.

Keep Tabs On Your Work

You can always keep a journal during your weight loss plan to help you figure out how well you are losing weight. This can include information on what you are eating, how you are exercising and so forth. This should help you understand what you can do when keeping yourself active.

Focus More On Control

While the goal here is indeed to lose weight, you have to especially think about your control and how long it is going to work for you. A great focus on control is important.
You have to think about how your weight loss plan is more of a plan for controlling your body. This is not so much about losing weight as it is for you to keep your body from gaining more weight than necessary. You have to be very cautious to ensure that you're not focused on just losing weight.
These mental strategies can make a real difference when used right. Make sure you think carefully about how you're going to go along with your weight loss goals so you won't struggle in the process of doing so.

Chapter 7 – Exercise Pointers

It's clear that you need to keep your body active if you want to lose weight. Exercise is a necessity for helping you to expend your energy stores so you will burn off fats the right way. You should prepare a sensible exercise routine to help you with your weight loss goals. This chapter is all about the types of exercises you can use to lose weight as well as what you should be doing to make your exercises more effective.

Cardio Workouts

Cardio, or cardiovascular, exercise is a popular form of exercise that can help you lose weight with ease. This is where you will work on movements that are fast and efficient and will help you to get your heart rate going.
Cardio workouts entail many things like:

- Running or jogging

- Swimming

- Climbing steps

- Bicycling

- Using an elliptical trainer

These are repetitive movements that improve how your heart functions and will cause you to use more energy. This in turn helps you to burn off fats with ease. This can be a great consideration for your workouts but you have to use a plan for cardiovascular exercise that is safe to handle.

Make sure you plan about 30 to 60 minutes of cardio workouts every other day. This will give you enough support for your body without forcing you to work any harder than necessary. It also gives you time to recover from the fatigue that may be caused by a workout.

Strength Training

Strength training is a solution to consider in that you can burn off your fats as they are converted into muscle mass. This works as the muscles will take in your calories and use them to expend energy. This in turn makes it to where your body will become stronger and capable of handling more weight. This can work with many exercises:

- Push-ups are great for the chest, arms and shoulders.

- Curl muscles are for the arms as you can move weights towards your body.

- Crunches are good to help strengthen your abdominal muscles.

- Leg presses can entail moving weights up and down with your feet.

Many of these exercises can work with your body providing the pressure and force. Sometimes added weights might be required but that will be optional in most cases.
Such exercises can work with as many repetitions as needed. You can always use about 10 to 15 repetitions of certain movements in a single set. This should be enough to give you enough time to build your muscles.

Aim to get about four or five days of strength training in with sessions going for about 15 to 20 minutes each time. A small amount of time is all you need as it not only improves upon your muscles but also keeps you from adding more weight than necessary.

Everyday Activities

Sometimes the everyday activities that you get into in your daily life can make a difference. You can use many daily activities to help you get yourself a little more energized while losing weight:

- A brisk walk can be taken in the morning to help you get ready for your day.

- Outdoor work like gardening and lawn care work can always help you stay active.

- See if there are any activities in your workplace that allow you to move around and do more work on the go. This is to ensure you don't just sit in one place during the entire working day.

No matter what you do, make sure you talk with a doctor to see what forms of exercise will work for you. Not all people are built to handle a variety of exercises. You have to ensure that your body can take in the pressure and effort needed for you to stay active and healthy.
Remember that your physical efforts will certainly make a difference when you're trying to stay healthy. The best exercises will help you lose weight but you should make sure it's kept under control and that you don't wear yourself out.

Chapter 8 – Important Lifestyle Changes

There are some essential lifestyle changes that also have to be made to ensure that you can lose weight properly. You must keep tabs on how you are living your life if you want to keep yourself from gaining weight or to at least keep your weight loss plans under control.

Creating Dietary Restrictions You Can Handle

It's a necessity to keep your diet from being worse than it could be. However, it is often a challenge for you to get rid of all that stuff you've been consuming for so long.
While it is best to avoid consuming harmful foods, you could instead create dietary restrictions that aren't as tough for you to handle as you might think they could be. For instance, you can start by drinking soda or alcohol on weekends instead of every day of the week.
A slight restriction in terms of what you are trying to consume will always be worthwhile. Over time you will begin to be less likely to want something that you had been dependent on. More importantly, you will start to notice that your body could feel a little more energetic and in control depending on whatever it is you are trying to get rid of.

Be Active During the Day

You should stay active during the day so you'll have more chances to lose weight. This comes from how you will move your body and put in more effort to help you stay ready for anything.
Here are a few things to do when looking to be active:
- Park further from the entrance to whether it is you work at when traveling to work.

- Use a bicycle to get around places instead of a car.

- Use the stairs instead of an escalator or elevator if you're able. You could always walk up or down an escalator too although you'd have to be cautious when getting on or off of it.

- It is better to walk to places than it is to use a moving walkway; this is a good point to use if you're ever at an airport.

Keep Your Body Hydrated

You must keep yourself hydrated at all times so you will have an easier time with keeping your body under control. You might need to get a few glasses of water in a typical day to keep yourself healthy.
You must keep plenty of water on hand throughout the day to keep you focused and to keep from having a desire to drink anything else. Water especially keeps you filled and could even boost metabolic processes as your body aim to heat itself up, thus burning fats in the process.

Use a Cold Shower

A great idea for your life is to use a cold shower every morning. A warm shower can open your pores and clean out dirt but it may actually be better for weight loss to go cold.
A cold shower will require your body to adjust its metabolic processes. This comes as the shower will trigger metabolism as the body aims to become warmer. This is in response to the tough cold weather that you might get into.

Substitute Foods Properly

You must also substitute the foods that you might normally consume properly. This includes the use of healthier foods that are easier for your body to handle. In particular, you can eat low-fat snacks like popcorn instead of some greasy potato chips.

You can also order a side salad to go with something you order at a restaurant instead of French fries or something that might be far too greasy. More places are willing to offer healthier concessions for your order so you'll have an easier time with managing your dietary needs as you are aiming to lose enough weight.

The key is to think about what types of foods are better for you and if you can handle them well enough. You might take a bit of time to get used to substituting different foods but it can make a real difference if you are careful enough and you know what you will get out of the process at large.

These lifestyle changes aren't all that hard for you to use when you understand how to make them work. It is amazing as to how easy it can be for you to lose weight if you are careful when doing so.

Conclusion

Weight loss isn't as hard to attain as you might think. You can easily lose weight when you use the right strategies for doing so. These great strategies will help you out by keeping your body from gaining weight while also triggering more weight loss functions as your metabolic functions keep working.

The points here are great to see as they entail the right foods to have in a 30-day period. These foods will keep you from having more fats in your body than needed. These also improve how well fat-burning processes can work.

When used with the right exercise plans and lifestyle changes, you will find it easy for you to lose weight. You can even add one of various different supplements to your body to help improve how well you can lose weight.

The results that you will get will vary based on how well you adhere to a weight loss plan. Fortunately, the process of doing so is so easy to handle that it should not be all that challenging for you to actually lose weight and keep it off.

Good luck with your weight loss endeavor. You will certainly be surprised when you take a look at the results you will get out of this weight loss plan.

www.ingramcontent.com/pod-product-compliance
Lightning Source LLC
Chambersburg PA
CBHW060442290526
45793CB00002B/540